BRAIN WASH COOKBOOK

Recipes that will help shape your cognitive health and make you cultivate a more purposeful and fulfilling life.

By

Kim Cox

The Brain Wash Cookbook

Copyright © 2020, By: *Kim Cox*

ISBN: 978-1-950772-74-2

All Rights Reserved. No part of this publication may be reproduced in any form or by any means, including scanning, photocopying, or otherwise without prior written permission of the copyright holder.

Disclaimer:

The information provided in this book is designed to provide helpful information on the subjects discussed. The publisher and author are not responsible for any specific health or allergy needs that may require medical supervision and are not liable for any damages or negative consequences from any treatment, action, application or preparation, to any person reading or following the information in this book.

The Brain Wash Cookbook

Table of Contents

INTRODUCTION: 6

Brain health recipes to help detox your mind for clearer thinking, deeper relationship and lasting happiness 6

The Brain Wash Recipes for a Healthy Brain 8

Mashed Banana & Whole-Grain Porridge 8

Very Blueberry Smoothie 10

Cranberry-Pumpkin Seed Energy Bars 11

Cranberry-Orange Spiced Oatmeal 13

Soba noodle & edamame salad with grilled tofu 15

Tofu & spinach cannelloni 17

Soy tuna with wasabi mash 19

Zingy salmon & brown rice salad 21

Salmon & soya bean salad 23

Edamame & chilli dip with crudités 25

Lemony three bean & feta salad 26

Tofu, greens & cashew stir-fry 28

Spicy tofu kedgeree 30

Quinoa tabbouleh 32

Waldorf slaw 33

Spaghetti with spinach & walnut pesto 34

Kale & apple soup with walnuts 35

Malted walnut seed loaf 37

Red cabbage with Bramley apple & walnuts 39

Late-summer tomato & carrot salad 41

Rainbow rice 42

Rapid rocket, carrot & ham salad 44

Steak & broccoli protein pots 45

Sesame salmon, purple sprouting broccoli & sweet potato mash 47

Poached eggs with broccoli, tomatoes & whole meal flatbread 49

Whole-wheat pasta with broccoli & almonds 51

Stir-fried chicken with broccoli & brown rice 53

Apple & blueberry Bircher 55

Chicken & avocado salad with blueberry balsamic dressing 56

Get up and go breakfast muffins 58

Instant frozen berry yogurt 60

Heart helper smoothie 61

Butternut soup with crispy sage & apple croutons 62

Pearl barley, parsnip & sage risotto 65

Salmon & spinach with tartare cream 67

Spring salmon with minty veg 69

Sticky salmon with Chinese greens 71

Super healthy salmon burgers 73

Salmon & ginger fish cakes 75

Hot-smoked salmon with creamy pasta & pine nuts 77

Salmon with warm chickpea, pepper & spinach salad 78

Marinated smoked salmon with poppy seeds 80

Rye & pumpkin seed crackers 82

Celeriac ribbons tossed with chard, garlic & pumpkin seeds 84

Raspberry and Blue Cheese Salad 86
Avocado and Orange Salad 87
Shrimp and Kiwi Salad 88
Pomegranate and Pear Jam 89
Lemon-Blueberry with Mascarpone Oatmeal 91
Grilled Mahi-mahi with Peach and Pink Grapefruit Relish .. 92
Tangerine and Avocado Salad with Pumpkin Seeds 94
Chipotle Pork and Avocado Wrap 95
Tomato-Basil Soup 97
Swiss Chard with Onions 98
Wilted Kale with Golden Shallots 99
Fennel Slaw with Orange Vinaigrette 100
Scandinavian salmon 102
Lemon vinaigrette dressing and salad 103
Vegetable soup served with brown rice 104

INTRODUCTION:

Brain health recipes to help detox your mind for clearer thinking, deeper relationship and lasting happiness

We all intuitively appreciate that the foods we consume shape our actions, thoughts, emotions and behavior. Most of the time we use food to soothe our moods and clear our heads without seeming to think much about it. The focus of most diets regime is on the way we look rather than the way we think. However, this is in part due to western society's fascination with appearance, and medicine's bias towards surgery and drugs. Contemporary medicine often disregards the ways that our diet helps shape our cognitive health and also medical students are not trained in nutrition.

In concrete terms, it entails that whatever you just ate will be part of what you will think. In the long term, this affects us all, because food affects not just our moods and thoughts but also the way we age with time. However, studies using next-generation imaging and genomic sequencing, both central to my work, have helped reveal that some foods such as fruit, wholegrains, vegetables, fish, nuts and seeds are neuro-protective. They do not only shield the brain from harm, but also support cognitive fitness over the course of a lifetime.

In fact, it comes perhaps as no surprise to us that other foods such as fried food, fast food, excess fatty foods and refined sugar are downright harmful instead, slowing us down, making us feel sluggish and tired, while at the same time deeply increasing our risk of dementia disease.

Research has shown that these effects are particularly evident by looking at brain scans of people on different diets. Let take this as an example, when we compared the scans of middle-aged people who had eaten a Mediterranean diet most of their lives with those of people of the same age who ate a western diet with processed food, processed meats, sweets and fizzy drinks, we saw the way the latter group's brains had shrunk prematurely. Subsequent studies provided even more heart troubling evidence that people on the western diet had started developing Alzheimer's plaques already in their 40s and 50s. Nevertheless, these are signs of accelerated ageing and increased risk of future dementia.

The foods we eat on regular basis can have a big impact on the structure and health of our brains. The brain is an energy-intensive organ, using around 20% of the body's calories, so it needs plenty of good fuel to maintain concentration all day long. Just as there is no magic pill to wipe off cognitive decline, no single almighty brain food can give you a sharp brain as you age. Nutritionists emphasize that the most necessary strategy is to follow a healthy dietary pattern that includes a lot of fruits, legumes, vegetables, and whole grains. You should try to get protein from plant sources and fish and choose healthy fats, such as olive oil or canola, rather than saturated fats.

Remember, a well-fed brain is one of your greatest assets when it comes to your career. Creating work, you're very proud of, thinking with a clear head, and communicating effectively are crucial to carving out your path and building your network. Not surprisingly, diet they say plays a starring role.

The bottom line is that the more processed, packaged and refined foods that you consume on a daily basis, the higher your risk of cognitive decline further down the line.

The Brain Wash Recipes for a Healthy Brain

Mashed Banana & Whole-Grain Porridge

Ingredients

- ¾ cup of mashed bananas
- Kosher salt
- Fresh fruit, toasted almonds and pure maple syrup (for serving)
- 2 cups of low-fat milk
- Pinch of ground cinnamon
- 4 cups of frozen mixed chewy grains (about 20 ounces), such as Kamut, wheat berries, barley and farro
- 2 tablespoons of quick-cooking oats

Directions:

1. First, in a medium saucepan, whisk the milk with the bananas, cinnamon and a generous pinch of salt.
2. After which you cook over moderate heat, stirring, until thickened slightly, about 3 minutes.

3. After that, add the frozen grains and oats and cook, stirring, until the grains are heated through and the porridge is creamy, about 5 minutes.
4. Then, spoon into bowls and top with fruit, almonds and maple syrup.

Make Ahead

NOTE: the porridge can be refrigerated overnight.

Make sure you reheat gently, adding milk as needed to thin out the porridge.

Very Blueberry Smoothie

Ingredients

- 2 cups of plain yogurt
- 1 cup of ice cubes
- 2 cups of fresh blueberries
- ¼ cup of milk
- 2 tablespoons of honey

Directions:

1. First, in a blender, combine the blueberries, milk, yogurt, and honey.
2. After which you puree until smooth.
3. Then, when ready to serve, add the ice and then pulse and blend the mixture until it is a smooth.
4. Finally, taste for sweetness and add more honey, if desired.

Cranberry-Pumpkin Seed Energy Bars

Ingredients

- 1 cup of rolled oats
- ¼ cup of flaxseeds
- ½ cup of honey
- ½ teaspoon of salt
- ½ cup of dried cranberries
- 1 cup of pecans (crushed)
- 1/3 cup of pumpkin seeds
- 2/3 cup of muscovado (or better still dark brown sugar)
- 4 tablespoons of unsalted butter
- 2 teaspoons of pure vanilla extract
- 2 cups of puffed rice cereal

Directions:

1. Meanwhile, heat the oven to 350° and line a baking sheet with parchment paper.
2. After which you spread the oats, pecans, pumpkin seeds and flaxseeds on the sheet and bake until fragrant, 8 minutes.
3. After that, transfer the mixture to a large bowl.

4. Then, in a saucepan, bring the sugar, honey, butter and salt to a boil over moderate heat.
5. At this point, simmer until the sugar is dissolved and a light brown caramel forms, 5 minutes.
6. This is when you remove from the heat and stir in the vanilla.
7. In addition, drizzle the caramel all over the nut-and-oat mixture. Stir in the puffed rice and cranberries until evenly coated.
8. After which you line an 8-inch square baking dish with parchment paper, extending the paper over the side.
9. Furthermore, scrape the cereal mixture into the dish in an even layer.
10. After that, cover the mixture with a second sheet of parchment and press down to compress it.
11. Then let stand until firm, about 2 hours.
12. At this point, discard the top piece of parchment.
13. Finally, using the overhanging paper, lift out the cereal square and transfer it to a work surface.
14. You can cut into 12 bars and serve.

Cranberry-Orange Spiced Oatmeal

Ingredients

½ teaspoon of ground cinnamon (or to taste)

½ cup of frozen blueberries

1 pinch of ground ginger (it is optional)

¼ cup of orange juice (or as needed)

¾ cup of old-fashioned rolled oats

¼ cup of dried cranberries

¼ teaspoon of ground turmeric (it is optional)

1 cup of water

Directions

1. First, place the rolled oats, cranberries, cinnamon, and blueberries in a microwave safe bowl.
2. After which you add the turmeric and ginger, if desired.
3. After that, pour in the water, and stir to mix ingredients.
4. At this point, cook on High until water is absorbed, about 2 minutes.

5. Finally, stir in orange juice to desired consistency.

Soba noodle & edamame salad with grilled tofu

Ingredients

300g fresh or preferably frozen podded edamame (soy) beans

300g bag beansprouts

250g block firm tofu (patted dry and thickly sliced)

Handful coriander leaves (to serve)

140g soba noodles

4 spring onions (shredded)

1 cucumber, peeled, halved lengthways, deseeded with a teaspoon and sliced

1 teaspoon oil

Ingredients for the dressing

2 teaspoons of tamari

1 red chilli (deseeded, if you like, and finely chopped)

3 tablespoons of mirin

2 tablespoons of orange juice

Directions:

1. First, heat dressing ingredients in your smallest saucepan, simmer for 30 secs, then set aside.
2. After which you boil noodles following the pack instructions, adding the edamame beans for the final 2 mins cooking time.
3. After that, rinse under very cold water, drain thoroughly and tip into a large bowl with the beansprouts, spring onions, cucumber, sesame oil and warm dressing (NOTE: season if you like).
4. At this point, brush tofu with the veg oil, season and griddle or grill for about 2-3 mins each side (NOTE: the tofu is very delicate so turn carefully).
5. Finally, top the salad with the tofu, scatter with coriander and serve

Tofu & spinach cannelloni

Ingredients

- 1 onion (chopped)
- 2 x 400g cans chopped tomatoes
- 400g bag of spinach
- 349g pack silken tofu
- 4 tablespoons of fresh breadcrumbs
- 2 tablespoons of olive oil
- 3 garlic cloves (finely chopped)
- 50g pine nuts (roughly chopped)
- Pinch grated nutmeg
- 300g pack fresh lasagna sheets

Directions:

1. First, heat half the oil in a pan, add onion and 1/3 of the garlic and fry for 4 mins until softened.
2. After which you pour in tomatoes, season and bring to the boil.
3. After that, reduce heat and cook for 10 mins until sauce thickens.
4. At this point, heat half remaining oil in a frying pan and cook another 1/3 of garlic for 1 min, then add half the pine nuts and the spinach.

5. This is when you wilt spinach, then tip out excess liquid.
6. Then, whizz tofu in a food processor or with a hand blender until smooth, then stir through the spinach with the nutmeg and some pepper.
7. Furthermore, remove from the heat; allow to cool slightly.
8. After that, heat oven to 200C/180C fan/gas 6.
9. After which you pour half tomato sauce into a 20 x 30cm dish.
10. In addition, divide spinach mix between lasagna sheets, roll up and lay on top of sauce.
11. At this point, pour over remaining sauce and bake for 30 mins.
12. Then, mix crumbs with remaining garlic and pine nuts.
13. Finally, sprinkle over top of dish, drizzle with remaining oil and bake for 10 mins until crumbs are golden.

Soy tuna with wasabi mash

Ingredients:

1 tablespoons of rice wine vinegar

2 tuna steaks (each about 140g/5oz)

100ml semi-skimmed milk

frozen broad bean (or better still soya beans, to serve)

3 tablespoons of soy sauce

1 tablespoon of caster sugar

500g potato

2 teaspoons of wasabi paste

1 spring onion (finely sliced)

Directions:

1. First, mix together the vinegar, soy sauce, and sugar.
2. After which you pour over the tuna and marinate for at least 20 mins or up to 2 hrs. in the fridge.
3. After that, place the potatoes in a pan of lightly salted boiling water, then cook for 10-15 mins until soft; Drain well.
4. Then, heat the milk in the pan and mix in the wasabi, return the potatoes to the pan, then mash until smooth.

5. At this point, stir through the spring onion and keep warm.
6. This is when you heat a non-stick griddle pan until smoking hot.
7. Furthermore, remove the tuna from the marinade.
8. After which you cook on the griddle for 2-3 mins on each side until seared on the outside, but still pink inside.
9. In addition, cook the broad or soy beans according to pack instructions, then serve alongside the tuna and mash.

Zingy salmon & brown rice salad

Ingredients

200g frozen soya beans (defrosted)

1 cucumber (diced)

Small bunch coriander (roughly chopped)

4 teaspoons of light soy sauce

200g brown basmati rice

2 salmon fillets

Small bunch spring onions (sliced)

zest and juice 1 lime

1 red chilli (diced, deseeded if you like)

Directions:

1. First, cook the rice following pack instructions and 3 mins before it's done, add the soya beans.
2. After which you drain and cool under cold running water.
3. In the meantime, put the salmon on a plate, then microwave on High for 3 mins or until cooked through.
4. After that, allow to cool slightly, remove the skin with a fork, then flake.
5. At this point, gently fold the spring onions, cucumber, coriander and salmon into the rice and beans.

6. Finally, in a separate bowl, mix the lime zest and juice, chilli and soy, then pour over the rice before serving.

Salmon & soya bean salad
Ingredients

200g frozen soya beans (defrosted)

2 tablespoons of flax seed oil (I prefer granoVita)

2 poached salmon fillets (skin removed)

1 large omega-3 rich egg

zest and juice 1 lemon

250g pouch Puy lentils

small bunch spring onions (sliced)

Directions:

1. First, put the egg in a pan, cover with cold water and bring to the boil.
2. After which you cook for 4 mins (or 8 for hard-boiled), adding soya beans to the pan for the final min, then drain and run under cold water to cool.
3. After that, shell and cut egg into 6 wedges, then set aside.
4. At this point, mix the lemon juice and zest with the oil, season, then stir through the soya beans, lentils and spring onions.
5. Finally, divide between 2 plates, then gently break the salmon into large flakes and put on top of the lentils along with

the egg. NOTE: try it with seeded brown bread.

Edamame & chilli dip with crudités

Ingredients

150g low-fat natural yogurt

juice 1 lime

handful coriander (chopped)

300g frozen soya bean

1 red chilli (chopped)

1 garlic clove (crushed)

1 red onion (finely chopped)

halved radishes, sticks of carrots, celery and peppers, to serve

Directions:

1. First, cook the soya beans in boiling salted water for 4 mins.
2. After which you drain and cool under cold running water.
3. After that, blitz with the yogurt, chopped red chilli, lime juice and crushed garlic clove until smooth.
4. Then, fold in the finely chopped red onion and a handful chopped coriander.
5. Finally, serve with halved radishes and sticks of carrots, celery and peppers.

NOTE: the dip will keep covered in the fridge for up to 3 days.

Lemony three bean & feta salad

Ingredients

200g frozen soya (or better still edamame beans)

½ red onion (finely chopped)

Pinch caster sugar

85g feta cheese (crumbled)

200g green bean (trimmed and halved lengthways)

400g can cannellini bean (drained and rinsed)

juice 1 lemon

1 teaspoon of poppy seed

Directions:

1. First, cook the green beans and edamame beans together in a pan of boiling water for 3 mins until tender.
2. After which you drain and cool under cold running water, then drain again and mix with the cannellini beans and red onion.
3. After that, add the sugar, lemon juice, poppy seeds and seasoning and stir through.

4. At this point, scatter the feta on top, then divide between plates or containers to pack into lunchboxes.

Tofu, greens & cashew stir-fry

Ingredients

- 1 head broccoli (cut into small florets)
- 1 red chilli (deseeded and finely sliced)
- 140g soya bean
- 2 x 150g packs marinated tofu pieces
- 25g roasted cashew nuts
- 1 tablespoon of vegetable oil
- 4 garlic cloves (sliced)
- 1 bunch spring onions (sliced)
- 2 heads Pak choi (quartered)
- 1 ½ tablespoons of hoisin sauce
- 1 tablespoon of reduced-salt soy sauce (feel free to add extra to suit your own taste)

Directions:

1. First, heat the oil in a non-stick wok.
2. After which you add the broccoli, then fry on a high heat for 5 mins or until just tender, adding a little water if it begins to catch.

3. After that, add the garlic and chilli, fry for 1 min, then toss through the spring onions, soya beans, Pak choi and tofu.
4. Then, stir-fry for about 2-3 mins.
5. Finally, add the hoisin, soy and nuts to warm through.

Spicy tofu kedgeree
Ingredients

- 1 onion (chopped)
- 2-3 pinches cayenne pepper
- 140g of basmati rice
- 1 red chilli (chopped)
- ½ bunch spring onions (sliced)
- 2 eggs
- 2 tablespoons of medium curry powder
- handful flat-leaf parsley (chopped)
- 1 tablespoon of olive oil
- 1 teaspoon of brown (or better still black mustard seeds)
- 100g marinated tofu (I prefer Cauldron)

Directions:

1. First, cook the rice and boil the eggs in the same pan for about 8-9 mins.
2. In the meantime, heat oil in a non-stick frying pan and soften the onion and chilli for 5 mins.
3. After which you add all the spices and fry for about 1-2 mins more.

4. After that, drain the rice and stir into the spicy onion with a splash of water and the tofu.
5. Then, season well, then heat through gently for a few mins until piping hot.
6. At this point, peel and quarter the boiled eggs.
7. Finally, stir the spring onions and parsley into the rice, divide between 2 bowls and top with the eggs.

Quinoa tabbouleh

Ingredients

- juice 1-2 lemons
- small bunch mint (chopped)
- bunch spring onions (sliced)
- handful walnuts (chopped)
- 200g quinoa
- 4 tablespoons of olive oil
- Small bunch flat-leaf parsley (chopped)
- ½ cucumber (deseeded and diced)

Directions:

1. First, rinse the quinoa well and place in a pan with about double the volume of water.
2. After which you bring to the boil, cover, reduce the heat and gently simmer for 10 mins or until the grain unwraps itself.
3. After that, turn off the heat and leave to cool slightly, then drain any remaining water.
4. Then, season the quinoa, stir in the lemon juice and oil and leave to cool fully.
5. Finally, stir in the other ingredients, then serve.

Waldorf slaw

Serves 6 - 8

Tip:

A wholesome, wintry salad recipe that makes the perfect side dish to ham or a pork pie

Ingredients

- 4 sticks celery (sliced)
- handful grapes (halved)
- 50g walnuts (roughly chopped)
- 1 small white cabbage (shredded)
- 2 green apples (peeled and diced)
- 6 tablespoons of light mayonnaise
- 1 tablespoon of white wine vinegar

Directions:

1. First, in a large bowl, combine the celery, cabbage, apples and grapes.
2. After which you mix the mayo with the vinegar and season.
3. After that, stir it into the vegetables so that they are well coated.
4. Then, sprinkle on the walnuts and serve. NOTE: will keep in the fridge for up to 3 days.

Spaghetti with spinach & walnut pesto

Ingredients

50g walnuts (roughly chopped)

Small punch parsley (roughly chopped)

350g whole-wheat spaghetti

100g bag baby spinach leaves

1 garlic clove (crushed)

Small bunch mint (roughly chopped)

zest and juice 1 lemon

50g raisins

Directions:

1. First, whizz the walnuts, garlic, herbs, lemon zest and juice with some seasoning in a food processor until finely chopped.
2. After which you cook the spaghetti following pack instructions, then drain reserving a little of the cooking water.
3. After that, return to the pan and stir in the pesto, raisins and spinach with a splash of cooking water.
4. Finally, serve with a drizzle of extra virgin olive oil, if you like.

Kale & apple soup with walnuts

Prep: 20 mins

Cook: 15 mins

Serves 2

Tip:

It is time to make the most of seasonal kale and give this soup added depth with sweet apple and a crunchy walnut topping - perfect as a healthy lunch

Ingredients

- 1 onion (finely chopped)
- 2 red apples (unpeeled and finely chopped)
- 500ml reduced-salt vegetable stock
- 20g pack of dried apple crisps (it is optional)
- 8 walnut halves (broken into pieces)
- 2 carrots (coarsely grated)
- 1 tablespoon of cider vinegar
- 200g kale (roughly chopped)

Directions:

1. **First, in** a dry, non-stick frying pan, cook the walnut pieces for 2-3 mins until toasted, turning frequently so they don't burn.

2. After which you take off the heat and allow to cool.
3. **After that, p**ut the carrots, onion, apples, vinegar and stock in a large saucepan and bring to the boil.
4. At this point, reduce the heat and simmer for 10 mins, stirring occasionally.
5. **Then, o**nce the onion is translucent and the apples start to soften, add the kale and simmer for an additional 2 mins.
6. Furthermore, carefully transfer to a blender or liquidizer and blend until very smooth.
7. Finally, pour into bowls and serve topped with the toasted walnuts, and a sprinkling of apple crisps, if you like.

Malted walnut seed loaf

Prep: 25 mins

Cook: 30 mins

Cuts into 12 thick slices

Ingredients

- 300g gluten-free brown bread flour (I prefer using Doves Farm)
- 85g potato starch
- 7g sachet easy-bake dried yeast
- 450ml milk (warmed to hand temperature)
- 1 tablespoon of white wine vinegar
- 50g walnut (roughly chopped)
- 100g corn flour
- 2 tablespoons of soya flour
- 2 teaspoons of xanthan gum
- 1 tablespoon of caster sugar
- 2 tablespoons of sunflower oil, plus extra for greasing
- 100g mixed seed (I prefer using linseeds, hemp seeds, pumpkin seeds and sesame seeds)

Directions:

1. First, mix the potato starch, yeast, flours, xanthan gum, sugar and 1½ teaspoon salt in a large bowl.
2. After which you mix together the milk, oil and vinegar in a separate bowl, then add to the dry ingredients and mix until a soft dough comes together.
3. After that, cover loosely with oiled cling film and leave to rise in a warm place for 1 hr.
4. Then, knead in most of the seeds and walnuts.
5. At this point, shape into a large round – oiled hands will help.
6. This is when you roll the round in the remaining seeds and nuts, then lift onto a baking tray.
7. Furthermore, loosely cover again with oiled cling film and leave for 1 hr. more.
8. After that, heat oven to 220C/200C fan/gas 7.
9. After which you bake the bread for 15 mins, then reduce oven to 190C/170C fan/gas 5 and continue baking for 30 mins until the loaf sounds hollow when tapped on the base.
10. Finally, leave on a wire rack to cool, wrapped in a clean tea towel – this will help to keep the loaf soft.

Red cabbage with Bramley apple & walnuts

Prep: 10 mins

Cook: 20 mins

Serves 8

Tip:

This recipe is a sweet, crunchy cabbage dish with a super healthy boost of vitamin C

Ingredients

- 25g butter
- 1 bay leaf
- 100ml cider vinegar
- Handful walnuts (toasted and chopped)
- 1 red cabbage (finely sliced)
- 1 Bramley apple (peeled and grated)
- 3 cloves
- 25g light muscovado sugar

Directions:

1. First, put the cabbage in a wide shallow pan with the apple, butter, bay leaf and cloves.
2. After which you cook, stirring, until the cabbage starts to wilt.
3. After that, add the vinegar (NOTE: stand back and don't breathe in until the steam

subsides), then continue to stir and cook until the vinegar has almost all disappeared.
4. Then, add the sugar and stir until it has completely dissolved (NOTE: be careful not to let it burn).
5. At this point, sprinkle with walnuts to serve.
6. Finally, this will freeze well but let it thaw completely before gently reheating in a pan or microwave.

Late-summer tomato & carrot salad

Ingredients

2 medium carrots (peeled and finely shredded or grated)

1 red chilli (deseeded and finely chopped)

2 tablespoons of balsamic vinegar

600g mixed ripe tomato, such as red and yellow cherry, plum and medium vine

Bunch spring onions (trimmed and finely chopped)

25g pumpkin seed

3 tablespoons of extra virgin olive oil

Directions:

1. First, chop the large tomatoes, halve the cherry ones and tip into a large serving bowl.
2. After which you add the spring onions, carrots, chilli and pumpkin seeds, and toss together.
3. After that, mix the extra virgin olive oil with the balsamic, a pinch of salt and a good grinding of black pepper.
4. Finally, pour over the tomatoes and toss together.

Rainbow rice

Prep: 10 mins

Cook: 20 mins

Tip:

This colorful salad recipe is a good way of getting lots of veggies and seeds into your children's diet

Ingredients

- 1 small red pepper (deseeded and finely chopped)
- 1 large carrot (grated)
- 2 tablespoons of toasted pumpkin seed or sunflower seeds
- ½ orange (juice only)
- 100g basmati rice, long grain rice or better still brown rice
- ½ cucumber (deseeded and finely chopped)
- 6 dried apricots (chopped)
- 2 tablespoons of olive oil

Directions:

1. First, cook the rice as per pack instructions.

2. After which you drain, rinse and drain again.
3. After that, mix with the cucumber, red pepper, grated carrot, dried apricots and toasted pumpkin seeds.
4. Finally, drizzle over olive oil and the orange juice.

Rapid rocket, carrot & ham salad

Ingredients

2 tablespoons of fresh orange juice

2 tablespoons of pumpkin seed

black pepper

1 large carrot

2 good handful of rocket

3-4 wafer thin slices lean ham

Directions:

1. First, coarsely grate the carrot and mix with the orange juice and some salt, if you want.
2. After which you mix the rocket with the pumpkin seeds.
3. Finally, top with lean ham and grind over some fresh black pepper.

Steak & broccoli protein pots

Prep: 10 mins

Cook: 9 mins

Serves 2

Tip:

This recipe is a tasty Japanese twist served with wholegrain rice and a zing of sushi ginger.

You can rustle them up in less than 20 minutes

Ingredients

- 2 tablespoons of chopped sushi ginger
- 225g lean fat-trimmed fillet steak
- 250g pack wholegrain rice mix with seaweed (Merchant Gourmet)
- 4 spring onions, the green part finely chopped, the white halved lengthways and cut into lengths
- 160g broccoli florets (cut into bite-sized pieces)

Directions:

1. First, tip the rice mix into a bowl and stir in the ginger, chopped onion greens and 4 tablespoons of water.

2. After which you add the broccoli and the spring onion whites, but keep the onions together, on top, as you will need them in the next step.
3. After that, cover with cling film, pierce with the tip of a knife and microwave for 5 mins.
4. In the meantime, heat a non-stick frying pan and sear the steak for 2 mins each side, then set aside.
5. Finally, take the onion whites from the bowl and add to the pan so they char a little in the meat juices while the steak rests.

Sesame salmon, purple sprouting broccoli & sweet potato mash

Prep: 10 mins

Cook: 15 mins

Serves 2

I think you should try this Asian-inspired salmon supper with a nutty sesame dressing, crisp veg and comforting sweet potato mash; it's healthy, low-calorie and rich in omega-3

Ingredients

1 tablespoon of low-salt soy sauce

1 garlic clove (crushed)

2 sweet potatoes (scrubbed and cut into wedges)

2 boneless skinless salmon fillets

1 red chilli, thinly sliced (deseeded if you don't like it too hot)

1 ½ tablespoons of sesame oil

Thumb-sized piece ginger (grated)

1 teaspoon of honey

1 lime (cut into wedges)

250g purple sprouting broccoli

1 tablespoon of sesame seeds

Directions:

1. First, heat oven to 200C/180 fan/ gas 6 and line a baking tray with parchment.
2. After which you mix together ½ tablespoon sesame oil, ginger, the soy, garlic and honey.
3. After that, put the sweet potato wedges, skin and all, into a glass bowl with the lime wedges.
4. Then, cover with cling film and microwave on high for 12-14 mins until completely soft.
5. In the meantime, spread the broccoli and salmon out on the baking tray.
6. At this point, spoon over the marinade and season.
7. Furthermore, roast in the oven for 10-12 mins, then sprinkle over the sesame seeds.
8. After that, remove the lime wedges and roughly mash the sweet potato using a fork.
9. In addition, mix in the remaining sesame oil, the chilli and some seasoning.
10. Finally, divide between plates, along with the salmon and broccoli.

Poached eggs with broccoli, tomatoes & whole meal flatbread

Prep: 5 mins

Cook: 6 mins

Serves 2

Tip:

With the protein-packed eggs with antioxidant-rich broccoli make this a healthy and satisfying breakfast choice

Ingredients

- 200g cherry tomatoes on the vine
- 2 whole meal flatbreads
- Good pinch of chilli flakes
- 100g thin-stemmed broccoli (trimmed and halved)
- 4 medium of free-range eggs (fridge cold)
- 2 teaspoons of mixed seeds (such as pumpkin, sunflower, sesame and linseed)
- 1 teaspoon cold-pressed rapeseed oil

Directions:

1. First, boil the kettle.

2. After which you heat oven to 120C/100C fan/gas 1/2 and put an ovenproof plate inside to warm up.
3. After that, fill a wide-based saucepan one-third full of water from the kettle and bring to the boil.
4. Then add the broccoli and cook for 2 mins.
5. At this point, add the tomatoes, return to the boil and cook for 30 secs.
6. This is when you lift out with tongs or a slotted spoon and place on the warm plate in the oven while you poach the eggs.
7. Furthermore, return the water to a gentle simmer.
8. After which you break the eggs into the pan, one at a time, and cook for 2 ½ - 3 mins or until the whites are set and the yolks are runny.
9. In addition, divide the flatbreads between the two plates and top with the broccoli and tomatoes.
10. After that, use a slotted spoon to drain the eggs, then place on top.
11. Then, sprinkle with the seeds and drizzle with the oil.
12. Finally, season with a little black pepper and the chilli flakes, and serve immediately.

Whole-wheat pasta with broccoli & almonds

Ingredients

1 red chilli, deseeded and sliced (feel free to add extra chilli if you like)

250g whole-wheat spaghetti

Zest one lemon

Parmesan shavings (or better still vegetarian alternative), to serve

2 tablespoons of extra-virgin olive oil

3 garlic cloves (thinly sliced)

300g thin-stemmed broccoli (cut into pieces)

25g flaked toasted almond

Directions:

1. First, bring a large pan of salted water to the boil.
2. In the meantime, heat the olive oil in a large frying pan.
3. After which you add the chilli and garlic, and cook on a low heat until golden.
4. After that, remove from the heat.
5. Then, add the pasta to the water and cook following pack instructions.
6. Furthermore, in the final 4 mins of cooking, add the broccoli.

7. After which once cooked, drain and tip into the garlic pan.
8. At this point, add the lemon zest and almonds, and toss together well.
9. Finally, serve in bowls, topped with Parmesan shavings.

Stir-fried chicken with broccoli & brown rice

Prep: 10 mins

Cook: 20 mins

Serves 2

Tip:

This is a combination of lean chicken with super-healthy broccoli, ginger and garlic for a quick and cheap, weeknight dinner

Ingredients

- 1 chicken breast (approx. 180g), diced
- 2 garlic cloves (cut into shreds)
- 1 roasted red pepper, from a jar (cut into cubes)
- 1 teaspoon of mild chilli powder
- 250g pack cooked brown rice
- 200g trimmed broccoli florets (about 6), halved
- 15g ginger (cut into shreds)
- 1 red onion (sliced)
- 2 teaspoons of olive oil
- 1 teaspoon of reduced-salt soy sauce
- 1 tablespoon honey

Directions:

1. First, put the kettle on to boil and tip the broccoli into a medium pan ready to go on the heat.
2. After which you pour the water over the broccoli then boil for 4 mins.
3. After that, heat the olive oil in a non-stick wok and stir-fry the ginger, garlic and onion for 2 mins, add the mild chilli powder and stir briefly.
4. Then, add the chicken and stir-fry for 2 mins more.
5. Furthermore, drain the broccoli and reserve the water.
6. At this point, tip the broccoli into the wok with the honey, soy, red pepper and 4 tablespoons of broccoli water then cook until heated through.
7. In the meantime, heat the rice following the pack instructions.
8. Finally, serve with the stir-fry.

Apple & blueberry Bircher

Prep: 10 mins

Serves 4

Tip:

This super healthy breakfast that's high in fiber and low in fat keeps your energy up all morning.

Ingredients

- ½ teaspoon of ground cinnamon
- 200g blueberries
- 200g porridge oats
- 500ml of apple juice
- 4 apples (grated)

Directions:

1. First, mix the porridge oats with the cinnamon in a large bowl.
2. After which you stir in the apple juice and grated apples, then gently fold in the blueberries.
3. Then allow to stand for 5 mins before serving, or leave overnight and enjoy for breakfast the next day.

Chicken & avocado salad with blueberry balsamic dressing

Prep: 15 mins

Cook: 5 mins

Serves 2

Tip:

This is a healthy, gluten-free dinner or lunch, perfect for using up leftover roast chicken. You can make it veggie by swapping the meat for a handful of pumpkin seeds.

Ingredients

- 85g blueberries
- 2 teaspoons of balsamic vinegar
- 1 large cooked beetroot (finely chopped)
- 175g cooked chicken
- 1 garlic clove
- 1 tablespoon of extra virgin rapeseed oil
- 125g fresh or frozen baby broad beans
- 1 avocado (stoned, peeled and sliced)
- 85g bag mixed baby leaf salad

Directions:

1. First, you finely chop the garlic.

2. After which you mash half the blueberries with the oil, vinegar and some black pepper in a large salad bowl.
3. After that, boil the broad beans for 5 mins until just tender.
4. Then, drain, leaving them unskinned.
5. At this point, stir the garlic into the dressing, then pile in the warm beans and remaining blueberries with the avocado, beetroot, salad and chicken.
6. Furthermore, toss to mix, but don't go overboard or the juice from the beetroot will turn everything pink.
7. Finally, pile onto plates or into shallow bowls to serve.

Get up and go breakfast muffins

Ingredients

- 150ml pot natural low-fat yogurt
- 100g apple sauce (or puréed apple)
- 4 tablespoons of honey
- 200g whole meal flour
- 1½ teaspoon of baking powder
- 1½ teaspoons of cinnamon
- 2 tablespoons of mixed seed I prefer using pumpkin, sunflower and flaxseed)
- 2 large eggs
- 50ml rapeseed oil
- 1 ripe banana (mashed)
- 1 teaspoon of vanilla extract
- 50g rolled oats (+ extra for sprinkling)
- 1½ teaspoon of bicarbonate of soda
- 100g blueberry

Directions:

1. First, heat oven to 180C/160C fan/gas 4.
2. After which you line a 12-hole muffin tray with 12 large muffin cases.

3. After that, in a jug, mix the yogurt, eggs, banana, apple sauce, oil, honey and vanilla.
4. Then, tip the remaining ingredients, except the seeds, into a large bowl, add a pinch of salt and mix to combine.
5. At this point, pour the wet ingredients into the dry, mix briefly until you have a smooth batter, don't over mix as this will make the muffins heavy.
6. This is when you spoon the batter between the cases.
7. Furthermore, sprinkle the muffins with the extra oats and the seeds.
8. After which you bake for 25-30 mins until golden and well risen, and a skewer inserted to the center of a muffin comes out clean.
9. Then, remove from the oven, transfer to a wire rack and leave to cool.
10. Finally, store in a sealed container for up to 3 days.

Instant frozen berry yogurt

Prep: 2 mins No cook

Serves 4

Tip:

Remember, 3 ingredients and two minutes is all you need to whip up this low-fat, low-calorie yogurt, which is ideal for eating after exercise

Ingredients

- 250g (0%-fat) Greek yogurt
- 1 tablespoon of honey or better still agave syrup
- 250g frozen mixed berry

Directions:

1. First, blend berries, yogurt and honey or agave syrup in a food processor for 20 seconds, until it comes together to a smooth ice-cream texture.
2. Then, scoop into bowls and serve.

Heart helper smoothie

Prep: 5 mins No cook

Serves 1

Ingredients

1 small apple (peeled, quartered and cored)

300ml water

2 small raw beetroots (peeled and roughly chopped)

50g blueberry

1 tablespoon of grated ginger

Directions:

First, put the apple, beetroot, blueberries and ginger in a blender, top up with water then blitz until smooth.

Butternut soup with crispy sage & apple croutons

Prep: 20 mins

Cook: 30 mins

Serves 4

Ingredients

1 large onion (chopped)

1 butternut squash, about 1kg (peeled, deseeded and chopped)

500ml gluten-free vegetable stock (plus a little extra if necessary)

sunflower oil (for frying)

1 tablespoon of olive oil

1 garlic clove (chopped)

3 tablespoons of madeira or dry Sherry

1 teaspoon of chopped sage, plus 20 small leaves, cleaned and dried

Ingredients for the apple croutons

1 large eating apple (peeled, cored and diced)

1 tablespoon of olive oil

A few pinches of golden caster sugar

Directions:

1. First, heat the oil in a large pan, add the onion and fry for 5 mins.
2. After which you add the garlic and squash, and cook for 5 mins more.
3. After that, pour in the Madeira and stock, stir in the chopped sage, then cover and simmer for about 20 mins until the squash is tender.
4. Then, blitz with a hand blender or in a food processor until completely smooth.
5. Furthermore, allow to cool in the pan, then chill until ready to serve. **NOTE:** will keep for 2 days or freeze for 3 months.
6. If you want to make the crispy sage, heat some oil (a depth of about 2cm) in a small pan, then drop in the sage leaves until they are crisp – you will need to do this in batches.
7. After which you drain on kitchen paper (**NOTE:** Will keep for several hours).
8. Just before serving, I suggest you reheat the soup in a pan.
9. At this point, the texture should be quite thick and velvety, but thin it with a little stock if it is too thick.
10. Furthermore, for the apple croutons, I suggest you heat the oil in a large pan, add the apple and fry until starting to soften.

11. This is when you sprinkle with the sugar and stir until lightly caramelized.
12. If you want to serve, ladle the soup into small bowls and top with the apple, sage and a grinding of black pepper.

Pearl barley, parsnip & sage risotto

Ingredients

1 onion (finely chopped)

1 garlic clove (crushed)

400g pearl barley (rinsed)

25g parmesan (or better still vegetarian alternative), grated, plus extra to serve

25g butter (+ an extra knob to stir through)

4 parsnips (about 500g, peeled and cut into chunks)

10 sage leaves (shredded, plus extra to serve)

1.4l hot vegetable stock

Directions:

1. First, heat the butter in a large saucepan.
2. After which you add the onion and a pinch of salt, and cook gently for 5 mins.
3. After that, tip in the parsnips, turn up the heat and cook for 8-10 mins, stirring every so often, until the parsnips are starting to brown and caramelise.
4. Then, add the garlic and sage, and mix through.

5. At this point, tip in the barley and stir to coat well.
6. This is when you pour in the stock, bring to the boil, then turn down to a simmer and cook for about 35-40 mins, or until nearly all the liquid has been absorbed and the pearl barley is tender but still has a bite. NOTE: you may need to add a little extra boiling water.
7. Furthermore, take off the heat, top with the Parmesan and a knob of butter, then leave to melt.
8. After which you give the risotto a good stir, then spoon into dishes.
9. Finally, top with more sage, Parmesan and some black pepper.

Salmon & spinach with tartare cream

Ingredients

2 skinless salmon fillets

2 tablespoons of reduced-fat crème fraiche

1 teaspoon of caper (drained)

Lemon wedges (to serve)

1 teaspoon of sunflower (or better still vegetable oil)

250g bag spinach

juice ½ lemon

2 tablespoons of flat-leaf parsley (chopped)

Directions:

1. First, heat the oil in a pan, season the salmon on both sides, then fry for 4 mins each side until golden and the flesh flakes easily.
2. After which you leave to rest on a plate while you cook the spinach.
3. After that, tip the leaves into the hot pan, season well, then cover and leave to wilt for 1 min, stirring once or twice.
4. Then, spoon the spinach onto plates, then top with the salmon.

5. At this point, gently heat the crème fraiche in the pan with a squeeze of the lemon juice, the capers and parsley, then season to taste. NOTE: be careful not to let it boil.
6. Finally, spoon the sauce over the fish, then serve with lemon wedges.

Spring salmon with minty veg

Ingredients

750g frozen pea and beans (I prefer using Waitrose pea and bean mix, £2.29/1kg)

Zest and juice of 1 lemon

4 salmon fillets about 140g/5oz each

750g small new potato (thickly sliced)

3 tablespoons of olive oil

Small pack mint (leaves only)

Directions:

1. **First, b**oil the potatoes in a large pan for 4 mins.
2. After which you tip in the peas and beans, bring back up to a boil, then carry on cooking for another 3 mins until the potatoes and beans are tender.
3. After that, whizz the olive oil, lemon zest and juice and mint in a blender to make a dressing (or finely chop the mint and whisk into the oil and lemon).
4. **Then p**ut the salmon in a microwave-proof dish, season, then pour the dressing over.
5. At this point, cover with cling film, pierce, then microwave on High for about 4-5 mins until cooked through.

6. Furthermore, drain the veg, then mix with the hot dressing and cooking juices from the fish.
7. Finally, serve the fish on top of the vegetables.

Sticky salmon with Chinese greens

Prep: 5 mins

Cook: 15 mins

Serves 4

Tip:

This is a quick way to liven up salmon fillets, with stir-fried veg and the classic trio of garlic, chilli and ginger

Ingredients

- 3 tablespoons of oyster sauce
- 1 tablespoon of honey
- 1 tablespoon of finely grated fresh root ginger
- 500g mixed green vegetables (I used book choi, sugar snaps and broccoli)
- 4 skinless salmon fillets (about 150g/4oz each)
- 2 tablespoons of teriyaki sauce
- 1 tablespoon of oil (a mix of vegetable and sesame)
- 1 garlic clove (finely sliced)
- 1 red chilli (deseeded and finely sliced)

Directions:

1. First, heat oven to 200C/fan 180C/gas 6.
2. After which you place the salmon on a baking tray.
3. After that, mix together the oyster sauce, teriyaki and honey, then brush a little over the fish.
4. Then, roast for about 8-10 mins until glazed and just cooked through; set aside.
5. At this point, heat the oil in a wok, then fry the ginger, garlic and chilli for 1 min.
6. Furthermore, stir-fry the broccoli or any larger, harder veg for 3 mins, then add the leafy veg and cook for 1-2 mins more.
7. Finally, stir in the rest of the sticky sauce, heat through and serve with the fish.

Super healthy salmon burgers

Ingredients

- 2 tablespoons of Thai red curry paste
- 1 teaspoon of soy sauce
- Lemon wedges (to serve)
- 4 boneless, skinless salmon fillets, about 550g/1lb 4oz in total, cut into chunks
- Thumb-size piece fresh root ginger (grated)
- 1 bunch coriander (half chopped, half leaves picked)
- 1 teaspoon of vegetable oil

Ingredients for the salad

- Half large or 1 small cucumber
- 1 teaspoon of golden caster sugar
- 2 carrots
- 2 tablespoons of white wine vinegar

Directions:

1. First, tip the salmon into a food processor with the paste, ginger, soy and chopped coriander.

2. After which you pulse until roughly minced.
3. After that, tip out the mix and shape into 4 burgers.
4. At this point, heat the oil in a non-stick frying pan, then fry the burgers for 4-5 mins on each side, turning until crisp and cooked through.
5. In the meantime, use a swivel peeler to peel strips of carrot and cucumber into a bowl.
6. Furthermore, toss with the vinegar and sugar until the sugar has dissolved, then toss through the coriander leaves.
7. Finally, divide the salad between 4 plates.
8. You can serve with the burgers and rice.

Salmon & ginger fish cakes

Prep: 15 mins

Cook: 30 mins

Serves 2

Ingredients

- 4 teaspoons of olive oil
- Thumbnail-size piece ginger (grated)
- 2 tablespoons of mayonnaise mixed with wasabi (optional)
- 1 large sweet potato (cut into chips)
- 2 x 140g/5oz skinless salmon fillets
- Zest 1 lime, + wedges to serve
- ½ bunch spring onions (finely chopped)

Directions:

1. First, heat oven to 200C/180C fan/gas 6.
2. After which you toss the chips in a roasting tin with 1 teaspoon oil.
3. After that, season and bake for 20-25 mins.
4. At this point, chop the salmon as finely as you can and place in a bowl with the ginger, lime zest and seasoning.

5. Then, heat 1 teaspoon oil in a non-stick pan and soften the spring onions for 2 mins.
6. Furthermore, stir into the salmon, mix well and shape into 4 patties.
7. After that, heat remaining oil in the pan and cook the patties for 3-4 mins each side until golden and cooked through.
8. Finally, cover with a lid and leave to rest for a few mins.
9. You can serve 2 patties each with the chips, mayo and lime wedges for squeezing.

Hot-smoked salmon with creamy pasta & pine nuts

Ingredients

100ml white wine

2 tablespoons of grated parmesan

85g toasted pine nut

600g trophy pasta

142ml pot double cream

450g hot-smoked salmon (skin removed and flaked into chunks)

Directions:

1. First, cook the pasta in boiling salted water according to pack instructions.
2. In the meantime, bring the wine to the boil in a large frying pan, then simmer for 1 min.
3. After which you reduce the heat, stir in the cream and season well.
4. Then, when the pasta is cooked, drain briefly and tip into the frying pan with the sauce.
5. Furthermore, add the Parmesan and flaked salmon pieces, and mix gently together.
6. Finally, pile into bowls, sprinkle with pine nuts and serve with the watercress salad (recipe below) alongside.

Salmon with warm chickpea, pepper & spinach salad

Prep: 5 mins

Cook: 15 mins

Serves 2

Tip:

Remember, this wholesome grilled salmon dish is ready in just 20 minutes but makes a smart meal for two

Ingredients

- Zest and juice ½ small lemon
- 1 tablespoon of extra-virgin olive oil
- 400g can chickpeas
- 1 large red pepper (quartered and deseeded)
- Pinch smoked paprika (I used sweet smoked paprika)
- 100g bag young leaf spinach
- 2 x 140g (about 2 x 5oz) skinless salmon fillets

Directions:

1. First, heat the grill.
2. After which you squash the pepper quarters flat and grill for 5 mins or until well blackened.

3. After that, leave the grill on, then transfer the peppers to a bowl, cover with cling film and leave to cool slightly before peeling off the skins and cutting the flesh into strips.
4. Then, make the dressing by whisking together the lemon zest, juice, smoked paprika, olive oil and seasoning.
5. At this point, toss half the dressing with the spinach leaves and divide between 2 bowls.
6. This is when you season the salmon and grill for 5 mins or until just cooked through.
7. In the meantime, heat the chickpeas in their canning liquid in a saucepan for 3-4 mins.
8. Furthermore, drain well, then mix with the remaining dressing and strips of pepper.
9. Finally, spoon over the spinach and top with the salmon to serve.

Marinated smoked salmon with poppy seeds

Prep: 15 mins No cook

Serves 6

Ingredients

- 2 oranges, zest of both, juice of 1
- 2 teaspoons of olive oil
- 300g of smoked salmon
- toasted rye or better still soda bread, to serve
- 1 tablespoon of poppy seed (lightly toasted)
- 2 teaspoons of red wine vinegar
- ½ teaspoon sesame oil
- 85g radish, trimmed and finely sliced
- 3 spring onions (finely sliced)

Directions:

1. First, whisk together the poppy seeds, orange zest and juice, vinegar and oils with some black pepper and a pinch of salt – be sparing with the salt, as smoked salmon is naturally quite salty.
2. After which you carefully separate the slices of salmon, then put into a mixing bowl with most of the radishes and spring onions.

3. After that, drizzle over the dressing and gently toss together lightly – using your hands is best.
4. Then, let the salmon marinate for just 5-10 mins while you toast the bread – any longer and the vinegar will begin to 'cook' the fish.
5. At this point, spread the salmon over a large plate or platter, pour over any dressing left in the bowl, then scatter over the reserved radishes and spring onions.
6. Finally, bring to the table with toasted bread and a few forks, and let everyone help themselves.

Rye & pumpkin seed crackers

Tip:

Remember, making your own crispbreads is an extra-special touch - top these seeded biscuits with pate, cheese and chutney

Ingredients

    200g whole meal flour

    ½ teaspoon of baking powder

    1 large egg

    200g rye flour

    100g pumpkin seed

    1 teaspoon of salt

    1 teaspoon of golden caster sugar

Directions:

1. First, heat oven to 140C/120C fan/gas 1 and line 2 baking trays with baking parchment.
2. After which you mix the dry ingredients in a large bowl.
3. After that, beat the egg with 250ml water in a jug, then pour into the dry mixture.
4. At this point, combine with a wooden spoon, then transfer to a lightly floured work surface and knead until you have a smooth, firm dough.

5. Furthermore, roll the dough out as thinly as possible and cut into squares, about 7cm.
6. This is when you transfer the squares to your baking trays.
7. After which you bake for 45 mins, then remove the trays from the oven.
8. In addition, flip each cracker over on the tray and return to the oven, swapping over the shelves, for a further 45 mins.
9. Then, once cooked, remove from the oven and transfer to a wire rack to cool.
10. Finally, store in a sealed container for up to 2 weeks.

Celeriac ribbons tossed with chard, garlic & pumpkin seeds

Ingredients

- 1 lemon, juiced
- 2 tablespoons of extra virgin olive oil
- 4 thyme sprigs (leaves removed)
- ½ teaspoon of dried chilli flakes
- 20g pecorino
- 1 small celeriac (peeled)
- 40g pumpkin seeds
- 15g butter
- 2 finely chopped cloves of garlic
- 1 bunch of chard, with leaves separated from stalks, stalks sliced and leaves shredded

Directions:

1. First, using a good vegetable peeler, cut long, wide strips (about the width of pappardelle) around the circumference of the celeriac, into a bowl of water and lemon juice, until you have lots of ribbons. A
2. After which you allow for more than you would if using pasta.

3. After that, dry-fry the pumpkin seeds in a pan until they've puffed and popped; set aside.
4. Then, bring a large pan of salted water to the boil.
5. Furthermore, add the celeriac for 1 min, drain and reserve the water.
6. At this point, in a non-stick frying pan, heat the oil and butter until the butter has melted and foamed up.
7. This is when you add the thyme, garlic and chilli.
8. In addition, cook the garlic mixture for 5 mins until fragrant and almost golden, add the chard stalks and stir, cooking for a couple more mins.
9. After that, add the pumpkin seeds and the chard leaves, season and squeeze in some lemon juice.
10. After which you turn up the heat and stir in half the grated cheese.
11. Then add the celeriac and a slosh of the cooking water and toss, shaking the pan until the sauce looks glossy.
12. Finally, divide between plates, top with more cheese and serve.

Raspberry and Blue Cheese Salad

Ingredients

1 ½ teaspoons red wine vinegar

1/8 teaspoon of salt

5 cups of mixed baby greens

1-ounce blue cheese

1 ½ tablespoons of olive oil

¼ teaspoon of Dijon mustard

1/8 teaspoon of pepper

½ cup of raspberries

¼ cup of chopped toasted pecans

Directions:

1. First, combine vinegar, salt, olive oil, Dijon mustard, and pepper.
2. After which you add mixed baby greens; toss.
3. Then top with raspberries, pecans, and blue cheese.

Avocado and Orange Salad

Ingredients

1 teaspoon of olive oil

¼ teaspoon of kosher salt

½ cup of halved grape tomatoes

1 cup of sliced avocado

1 tablespoon of minced garlic

½ teaspoon of black pepper

1 orange

¼ cup of thinly sliced red onion

Directions:

1. First, combine olive oil, garlic, black pepper, and kosher salt in a medium bowl.
2. After which you peel and section orange; squeeze membranes to extract juice into bowl.
3. After that, stir garlic mixture with a whisk.
4. Then, add orange sections, onion, grape tomatoes, and avocado to garlic mixture; toss gently.

Shrimp and Kiwi Salad
Ingredients

12 peeled and deveined large shrimp (about 3/4 pound)

1 tablespoon of chopped fresh cilantro

1 tablespoon of fresh lime juice

1/8 teaspoon salt

1/8 teaspoon of black pepper

1 cup of cubed peeled kiwifruit (about 3 kiwifruit)

1 tablespoon of olive oil (divided)

1 tablespoon of chopped green onions

1 tablespoon of rice vinegar

1 teaspoon of grated lime rind

1/8 teaspoon of crushed red pepper

2 cups of torn red leaf lettuce leaves

Directions:

1. First, heat 1 teaspoon oil in a large nonstick skillet over medium-high heat.
2. After which you add shrimp; sauté 4 minutes or until done.
3. Then, remove from heat.

Pomegranate and Pear Jam

Ingredients

2 cups of chopped, peeled Seckel (or other) pear

¼ cup of rose wine

½ teaspoon of butter

1 teaspoon of minced fresh rosemary

2 cups of sugar

2/3 cup of strained fresh pomegranate juice (about 2 pomegranates)

¼ cup of pomegranate seeds

2 tablespoons of fruit pectin for less- or no-sugar recipes (such as Sure-Jell in pink box)

1 tablespoon of grated lemon rind

Directions:

1. First, combine pear, sugar, pomegranate juice, and wine in a large saucepan over medium heat; stir until sugar melts.
2. After which you bring to a simmer; simmer 25 minutes or until pear is tender.
3. After that, remove from heat; mash with a potato masher.
4. Then, add pomegranate seeds and butter; bring to a boil.
5. At this point, stir in fruit pectin.
6. This is when you return mixture to a boil; cook 1 minute, stirring constantly.

7. Furthermore, remove from heat; stir in lemon rind and rosemary.
8. Finally, cool to room temperature.
9. You can cover and chill overnight.

Lemon-Blueberry with Mascarpone Oatmeal

Ingredients

½ cup of old-fashioned oats

1 teaspoon of sugar

3 tablespoons of fresh blueberries

2 teaspoons of sliced toasted almonds

¾ cup of water

Dash of salt

1 tablespoon of prepared lemon curd

1 teaspoon of mascarpone cheese

Directions:

1. First, bring water to a boil in a medium saucepan.
2. After which you stir in oats and dash of salt.
3. After that, reduce heat; simmer 5 minutes, stirring occasionally.
4. Then, remove from heat, and stir in sugar and lemon curd.
5. Finally, top oatmeal with mascarpone cheese, blueberries, and almonds.

Grilled Mahi-mahi with Peach and Pink Grapefruit Relish

Ingredients

2 tablespoons of brown sugar

2 ½ cups of diced peeled ripe peaches (about 1 ½ pounds)

1/2 cup of small mint leaves

6 (6-ounce) mahi-mahi or other firm whitefish fillets (about 3/4 inch thick)

1/3 cup of rice vinegar

½ cup of finely chopped red onion

1 ½ cups of pink grapefruit sections (about 2 large grapefruit)

¾ teaspoon of salt (divided)

½ teaspoon of black pepper (divided)

Direction:

1. First, prepare grill.
2. After which you place vinegar and sugar in a small saucepan; bring to a boil.
3. After that, remove from heat.
4. Then, place onion in a large bowl.
5. At this point, pour vinegar mixture over onion, tossing to coat; cool.
6. This is when you add grapefruit, mint, peaches, ¼ teaspoon salt, and ¼ teaspoon pepper to onion; toss gently.

7. Furthermore, sprinkle fish with ½ teaspoon salt and ¼ teaspoon pepper.
8. Finally, place fish on grill rack coated with cooking spray; grill 5 minutes on each side or until fish flakes easily when tested with a fork.

Tangerine and Avocado Salad with Pumpkin Seeds

Ingredients

1 small avocado (peeled and sliced)

1 teaspoon of extra-virgin olive oil

Dash of kosher salt

2 tangerines (peeled)

1 tablespoon of fresh lime juice

3 tablespoons of toasted pumpkin seeds

¼ teaspoon of chili powder

Directions:

1. First, cut tangerines into rounds.
2. After which you combine avocado, tangerines, lime juice, and olive oil; toss gently to coat.
3. Then, sprinkle with pumpkin seeds, chili powder, and a dash of kosher salt.

Chipotle Pork and Avocado Wrap

Ingredients

1 ½ tablespoons of low-fat mayonnaise

2 teaspoons of chopped canned chipotle chiles in adobo sauce

¼ teaspoon of ground cumin

4 (8-inch) fat-free flour tortillas

¼ cup of bottled salsa

½ cup of mashed peeled avocado

1 teaspoon of fresh lime juice

¼ teaspoon of salt

¼ teaspoon of dried oregano

1 ½ cups (1/4-inch-thick) slices cut Simply Roasted Pork (about 8 ounces)

1 cup of shredded iceberg lettuce

Directions:

1. First, combine the avocado, low-fat mayonnaise, fresh lime juice, chipotle chiles in adobo sauce, salt, ground cumin, oregano, stirring well.
2. After that, warm tortillas according to package directions.
3. At this point, spread about 2 tablespoons avocado mixture over each tortilla, leaving a 1-inch border.

4. Then, arrange Simply Roasted Pork slices down center of tortillas.
5. Finally, top each tortilla with ¼ cup shredded lettuce and 1 tablespoon salsa, and roll up.

Tomato-Basil Soup
Ingredients

3 garlic cloves (minced)

¾ teaspoon salt

Basil leaves (it is optional)

2 teaspoons of olive oil

3 cups fat-free, less-sodium chicken broth

3 (about 14.5-ounce) cans no-salt-added diced tomatoes, undrained

2 cups of fresh basil leave (thinly sliced)

Directions:

1. First, heat oil in a large saucepan over medium heat.
2. After which you add garlic; cook 30 seconds, stirring constantly.
3. After that, stir in the broth, salt, and tomatoes; bring to a boil.
4. Then, reduce heat; simmer 20 minutes; Stir in basil.
5. At this point, place half of the soup in a blender; process until smooth.
6. Furthermore, pour pureed soup into a bowl, and repeat procedure with remaining soup.
7. Finally, garnish with basil leaves, if desired.

Swiss Chard with Onions
Ingredients

2 cups of thinly sliced onion

1 teaspoon of Worcestershire sauce

1/8 teaspoon of black pepper

2 teaspoons of olive oil

8 cups of torn Swiss chard (about 12 ounces)

¼ teaspoon of salt

Directions:

1. First, heat oil in a large nonstick skillet over medium-high heat.
2. After which you add onion; sauté 5 minutes or until lightly browned.
3. After that, add chard; stir-fry 10 minutes or until wilted.
4. Then, stir in Worcestershire, salt, and pepper.

Wilted Kale with Golden Shallots

Ingredients

2 sliced shallots

¼ teaspoon of salt

2/3 cup of unsalted chicken stock

2 tablespoons of olive oil

8 cups of lacinato kale (stemmed and chopped)

¼ teaspoon of black pepper

Directions:

1. First, heat a Dutch oven over medium heat.
2. After which you add olive oil; swirl to coat.
3. After that, add sliced shallots; cook 5 minutes or until golden, stirring frequently.
4. Then you add kale, salt, and pepper to pan; cook 2 minutes.
5. Finally, add chicken stock; cover and cook 4 minutes or until tender, stirring occasionally.

Fennel Slaw with Orange Vinaigrette
Ingredients

1 tablespoon of sherry vinegar

1 ½ tablespoons of fresh orange juice

¼ teaspoon of freshly ground black pepper

3 medium fennel bulbs with stalks (about 4 pounds)

½ cup of coarsely chopped pitted green olives

¼ cup of extra-virgin olive oil

1 teaspoon of grated orange rind

1 teaspoon of kosher salt

¼ teaspoon of crushed red pepper

2 cups of orange sections (about 2 large oranges)

Directions:

1. First, combine the first 7 ingredients in a large bowl.
2. After which you trim tough outer leaves from fennel; mince feathery fronds to measure 1 cup.
3. After that, remove and discard stalks.
4. Then, cut fennel bulb in half lengthwise; discard core.
5. Thinly slice bulbs and add fronds, fennel slices, and orange sections to bowl; toss gently to combine.

6. Finally, sprinkle with olives.

Scandinavian salmon

Prep: 5 minutes

Cook: 15 minutes

Ingredients (serves 4)

½ cup of water

1 tablespoon butter (softened)

1 small garlic clove (minced)

4 teaspoons of salmon roe (it is optional)

½ cup of dry white wine

4 salmon fillets (about 80g each)

1 teaspoon of chopped parsley

Salt (to taste)

Directions

1. First, heat wine and water over medium high heat in a large non-stick pan (approx. 5 minutes).
2. After which you slide salmon pieces into poaching liquid and dot with butter.
3. After that, sprinkle with dried parsley, garlic, and salt to taste.
4. Then, bring to a slow boil, reduce heat to medium and poach until salmon flesh is firm, about 10 minutes.
5. Finally, plate and sprinkle with salmon roe (optional)

Lemon vinaigrette dressing and salad

Ready in: 5 minutes

Ingredients (serves 4)

4 tablespoons of extra virgin olive oil

Selection of broccoli sprouts, baby greens, and cherry tomatoes

Juice of one lemon

2 tablespoons of balsamic vinegar

1 tablespoon of maple syrup (optional)

Directions:

1. First, put all ingredients into a small jar and mix to combine.
2. Then, pour over the mixed salad.

Vegetable soup served with brown rice

Prep: 20 minutes (NOTE: less than 10 minutes if using an electric chopper)

Cook: 25 minutes

Ingredients (serves 6 or more)

1 cup red cabbage (finely chopped)

6 medium carrots (finely chopped)

4 stalks of organic celery (finely chopped)

2 cups of sweet peas (frozen are good)

3cm piece ginger root (grated)

Brewer's yeast, 1 teaspoon per person

450g broccoli (finely chopped)

1 small onion (chopped)

6 green onions (finely chopped)

4 cloves of garlic (finely chopped)

1 cup of shelled edamame (e.g. soybeans)

3 liters of vegetable broth (no added salt)

2 tablespoons of extra virgin olive oil

Directions

1. First, put all the veg in a large pot.

2. After which you add broth and bring to a boil.
3. After that, cover and simmer for 20 minutes or until tender. (NOTE: Personally, I prefer to cook these al dente as I prefer the consistency better than mushy vegetables and I believe it preserves the veggies' ability to better deliver nutrients).
4. Then, turn off the heat, add olive oil and let cool for a few minutes.
5. At this point, distribute in bowls.
6. Furthermore, sprinkle brewer's yeast over the soup.
7. Finally, add brown rice for extra texture.